THIS ISN'T THERAPY

THIS ISN'T THERAPY

A Tough Love Approach to Living a Better Life

CHAZ MALEWSKI

CONTENTS

One
The Three Stages of Change   14

Two
Comfortably Uncomfortable   25

Three
Audit Your Life   34

Four
The Only 3 Things Keeping You From Change   48

Five
The Core Principles of Change   63

Six
Principle 1: No One Is Coming To Save You   68

Seven
Principle 2: One Percent   78

Eight
Principle 3: D.C.A (Decide. Commit. Act.)   87

Nine
Principle 4: Prioritize Growth   96

Ten
The Biggest Lie You Tell Yourself   106

Eleven
Shedding Skin   112

Want More?   119

Introduction

Picture this if you will......

You've come to the end of your life. The blinding LED light of the hospital room is the only thing indicating you're still here and not in the great beyond.

The bed is stiff against your back. You try to remember what your own bed feels like but you have no idea how long it's been since you've been home.

The tubes helping you breathe are irritating your throat and nasal passageways. The numbing agents being pumped into your system are doing their best to ease the inevitable. It feels as though you're being kept alive long enough to die.

All food tastes like mushy chalk. That is, when you're hungry enough to even eat any of it.

The room is cold and dry. You can't get comfortable no matter how many times you shift your body. The bed sores have slowly started working their way up your legs and onto your back.

You're too weak to speak. Otherwise you'd be asking for some help. Or some water.

And as you lay miserable in your hospital bed coming to grips with your reality, you take a moment to acknowledge the fear you've been running from for what feels like your whole life.

You're dying

Hours go by and familiar faces start piling in to see your not-so-smiling, tube-filled, pale face.

You're surrounded by your loved ones, friends and family; all nervously awaiting your passing. Everyone is stifling their emotions long enough to force a smile as they grab at your hands, arms, legs, toes...everything.

They shower you with praises and well wishes for a speedy recovery. They comment on how nice your room is and how good your food looks. All of them just trying to provide you with some small feeling of comfort. Little do they know you can barely make out what any of them are saying.

Even still, in this moment of silent agony, you feel a wave of comfort wash over you as you allow yourself a moment to soak in their presence one last time.

You know this is it; this is the end. But you don't want to say goodbye.

You try to hold their hands and tell them you love them, but the oxygen tubes have dried you out so much you can't say a single word. So you open your mouth and let out a small gasp; It's the best you can do.

Your skin has gone numb from the pain medications coursing through you, so you can't feel anyone's touch.

As the crowd of family and friends say their final goodbyes, you realize upon the closing of the hospital room door that you are truly alone. The only person in that room is *you*.

Left to die.

Alone.

And as you lie there waiting for your proverbial clock to stop ticking, you begin to think.

You begin to think about what's to come. What lies ahead for you in the great unknown? What legacy will you leave behind once you're gone? Will it hurt? Will you finally feel peace?

Your mind races to a million scenarios, each one more terrifying than the next. You realize your mind is spinning out of control and your heart begins to race. You hear the beeping of your heart rate monitor increase in volume and speed.

You know if the monitor gets too high of a reading, the nurse will come in and give you more medication. You're done with the medication. You just want to feel ok.

So, in a desperate attempt at lowering your heart rate, you think back on your life.

And as you drift off into thought, you realize you've never really taken the time to reflect on your life. You've always carried an "It is what it is" mentality and let your life just....happen.

You begin feeling something you can't quite describe; Something you've avoided all these years.

And that's when you feel the regret.

You're too weak to push the pain away this time. Reality has forced its hand.

- You remember that time you were on the fence about starting your own business and decided to stay in your unfulfilling corporate job. You kept telling yourself it was "only going to be another year." And then one year turned to 50.

- You remember not wanting to take the risk on that relationship you knew felt right for you and as a result, you suffered multiple divorces with the wrong people.

- You remember making excuses for being overweight and, as a result, you didn't have the energy to play and spend quality time with your kids after work. Now all you want is one more day with them.

Your memories begin to spiral into the pain of regret. You no longer feel any of the physical pains associated with your hospital treatment - all you can focus on is what you wish you would have done differently.

The emotions are almost overwhelming as you recount every risk you didn't take and the life you lived as a result of each one of those missed opportunities.

You're taken with an overwhelming yearning to go back and change your past mistakes. You begin to beg for more time, "PLEASE! Just give me one more chance!"

You want to jump out of bed and take back control of the life you let slip by. You want to live!

You frantically pull at the tubes and wires connected to you, alerting the medical staff that something is wrong. You're just trying to break free.

You struggle to sit up in the bed and immediately fall back, feeling dizzy from the sudden shift in blood flow.

Concerned, fuzzy faces of medical personnel rush in checking your vitals and machine readings. They ask if you want more pillows to help with comfort.

You feel powerless and angry. You can't speak. You can't move. You can't eat.

The only choice you have in this moment is to stay alive long enough to spite death. So you attempt once more to break free from the confines of your partially elevated hospital bed.

But the more you resist, the faster it takes you.

Minutes crawl by as you feebly attempt to lift your arms and remove your oxygen tubes. You burnt up all your energy on your previous escape attempt.

You realize this is it. This is truly the end.

No more opportunities. No more second-chances. No more "I'll start on Monday."

No more.

You stare, broken and defeated, up at the ceiling.

Your breathing slows.

The LED's start to dim.

You feel a tear slide slowly out of the corner of your eye.

And you die.

* * *

For some of you, this book is a guide. An instruction manual to an entirely different life. A code of being for the duration of your personal development journey. A way out of pain.

For some of you, this book is a warning. A warning of what's to come if you don't change. A caution sign on a slippery road. A notice of "attention, attention."A wake up call.

For all of you...

This Isn't Therapy.

* * *

I'd love to say this is going to be like every other personal development book you'd find on Amazon or your local bookstores.

You know the ones...

The books with the semi-confident coach leaning to the side like, "Hey, I'm just one of you guys!" Usually they have a sunset background or some other image meant to calm you.

Or maybe one of those ambiguous "The Secret to Everlasting Change and Happiness" books with an abstract image on the cover of an apple rolling off a table creating questions in your mind as to why that image is even relevant to the book.

Look, what I'm saying here is that there are a *ton* of self-help and personal development books available for purchase, and most of them are the same or extremely similar.

And, let's be honest, most of the content is just a regurgitated version of the last five personal development books you read. All promising to be "the last" solution you'll ever need to any of your life's problems.

Now, as with all things in this life, there are exceptions to the rule. I think if those books help you then you should read every single one. I've read many myself!

In fact, that's one of the pieces early on in my life that got me interested in the personal development field in the first place - reading those cheesy books!

But sometimes, positive thinking isn't enough. Sometimes, you just need someone to pull your eyes open, show you the path forward and say, "Walk."

Which is why I wrote This Isn't Therapy.

This is not your typical "feel good" self-help book.

You won't find any fluff or filler inside. I don't find that to be the best use of our time and, if you're taking the time to read this, I want you to get massive value out of every single page.

I wrote this book for a *very* specific reason.

It's meant to change you. And it's meant to change you for good.

Once you read this, there's no turning back. The guiding life change principles you'll learn in this book will stick to the back of your mind like gum on a shoe.

You won't be able to ignore them.

And that's the point...

When I got started in my own personal development journey, I had no idea what I really hoped to get out of it. I thought I would just get a few doses of motivation coupled with a spiritual element like meditation or hypnosis.

It wasn't until I started on my own *deep* work and started diving down into reasons I behaved the way I behaved in the past did I start to realize what this was all about. I started learning my own repetitive patterns that I did every day without even noticing that had been limiting me from hitting any significant goal. I learned about my ego and how it was practically controlling my mind to protect myself from admitting I was wrong. I cried for the first time in years. I felt like I was finally learning who *I* was, not just who everyone else wanted me to be. I felt alive. I felt free.

Free from the torment of never feeling like I was good enough in anything that I did. Free from the need to explain myself or my actions to others for fear of rejection. Free from the need to be "right" all the time and more accepting of other viewpoints or opinions. **I was free from the burdens the old me carried for so many years.**

So, naturally, I consumed every piece of personal development materials I could get my hands on:

- Books

- Videos

- Audio Programs

- Podcasts

- Seminars

- Courses

The list itself could be a book.

But after a while, I started to notice a trend with all of these personal development tools.

They all started to sound the same. They all taught similar lessons and gave the same, generic "This is how you change your life!" advice.

And every time I'd read/watch/attend anything personal development related, I'd feel a surge of motivation.......

......and then do nothing.

So, when I finally took time to reflect on everything I'd learned and what I'd started putting into practice, I noticed the most important piece of my growth journey thus far:

None of these books, podcasts, seminars, etc. were *pushing* me. They were making me feel good - read: distracted - in the moment, but none of them took me head on, challenged my self-imposed limits, and dared me to try harder.

I hired a life coach in 2014 and he pushed me to grow harder than I've ever been encouraged to by any coach, teacher, professor, etc. And my life transformed in front of me seemingly over a period of a few months. That's when I knew what I wanted my mission to be in this life.

I committed, from that moment on, to give that gift - that PUSH - to everyone that I possibly could.

I push my clients to grow harder than they've ever grown before. I challenge them. I call them to level up even when they don't see it as possible. I help them believe in themselves and actually do something about it. I give them what they'll never have in an inspirational book/movie/seminar.

And *that's* why I wrote this book.

I want this to be the last personal development book you ever read. And yes, you *need* to read it. Think of every other book like this you bought, read a little portion of, and then set it on a shelf only to think about it right now as I'm calling you out.

Don't start this reading journey the same way you've started with all the others. You can't create a new cycle by repeating the old one.

Inside you will find a few chapters pre-framing the reading experience and opening your eyes to some new insight. You'll start drawing some parallels to your own life and you'll start to understand yourself at a much deeper level than ever before.

You'll learn why you do the things you do, why you feel the things you feel, and why - despite your best efforts - you still feel stuck.

The core of this book contains 4 guiding principles that, if applied, will change your life.

Here's why:

This book will make you uncomfortable.

It will frustrate you.

It will poke around in those dark corners of your mind that you've worked so hard to hide.

It will fight your natural reaction to resist and run away.

It will make you think very hard at times.

It will make you address your demons.

It will (probably) make you cry.

It will call you to take action.

And as a result...

Your life will change.

But only if you read it and apply what you read.

I wrote this book for **you**. Let's get started.

-Chaz

CHAPTER ONE

The Three Stages of Change

"We are taught you must blame your father, your sisters, your brothers, the school, the teachers - but never blame yourself. It's never your fault. But it's always your fault, because if you wanted to change you're the one who has got to change."

-Katharine Hepburn

Many of you reading this right now are totally unaware, but you're already in the first stage of change - *awareness.*

You're aware that something in your life is not the way you want it to be, so you've decided to read this book in hopes of finding the solution.

For some of you, this is a massive step forward - congratulations!

For others, this is another attempt at finally building the life you want as opposed to settling into the life you have. You also deserve recognition.

Whatever brings you here, I want you to know you're meant to be here. You're meant to change.

And all change starts with awareness.

If we're going to make any form of meaningful, lasting change we have to know what we're changing and *why*.

The "why" is the most important part.

It's the driver. The motivator. The persistent voice in your head that tells you to keep going when life starts throwing punches.

If you don't have a strong reason for "why" you want to change, then you'll fall short of your goals every time. Because what's the point?

If you changed just because you kinda sorta wanted to be different, there would be no emotional attachment to the outcome. Same reasoning applies if your reason for changing is to make someone else happy.

It would be like getting dressed to go to a party that you reluctantly said yes to, only to feel relieved when you get the text message saying plans fell through and the party was off. Oh well, on with your life.

If change doesn't inspire you, change won't happen.

Which brings us knee bent and chin raised to our first stage of change:

1. AWARENESS

One day we wake up and we notice we gained a few pounds...

We start to notice our attitude has been getting increasingly negative over the years...

We start blaming other people for things that are happening to us instead of taking action to correct them...

Days turn to weeks and we realize we've let our lives slip into autopilot without even realizing.

This is what we call becoming *painfully aware.*

Awareness is the most uncomfortable stage of change, which is why most of us ignore admitting the truth about our situation and tell ourselves convenient little lies like:

"It's not that bad"

"I've been worse"

"I'm working on it"

"When I have (x), then I'll be ready"

These micro-excuses lead to macro-problems if left unchecked long enough.

Which is why it's now your turn for some (loving) painful awareness.

The number one change I want to make in my life is:

_____

I want to make this change because:

(**HINT**: this is your why)

_____

Now, celebrate!

You just took a step that most people wait far too long, if at all, to take. You became aware of what needs to change.

Now, before you go screaming from the rooftops, there's something you need to know.

Awareness is a trickster.

See, awareness would have you believe that now that you've identified what needs to change, you've made progress.

While on an extremely small scale you've made progress mentally, it translates very little to real world results.

Because awareness is just the first step of walking through the stages of change. If you stop at awareness, you'll be no better off than you were before other than knowing the truth of your situation.

Which is why we have to move to our second and most fundamental stage of change:

2. WILLINGNESS

Awareness is great, but if you're not willing to make the change, you'll always find a way to slip into your comfort zone and risk very little (more on this next chapter).

Willingness is the most difficult stage of change because it carries with it the risk of loss.

When you become willing to make changes in your life, that means you're willing to forego the things you already have and hold dear that are preventing you from moving forward.

This may translate to:

- Less time with friends and family.
- Increased stress.
- Becoming vulnerable.
- Asking for help.
- Spending money.
- Looking dumb in front of your peers.
- Risk of failure.
- Risk of success.

- Etc.

There is a weight to willingness that can only be sufficiently carried by those with a strong enough reason why. Which is why I had you write yours out earlier.

Speaking of...

Now that you know the weight of willingness, is your why strong enough to carry you through or do you need to go back and rewrite it?

Because willingness also likes to play a game with you. Willingness pushes you to make a decision. And when your decision is made, it feels like the stars align and you're all of a sudden moving at light speed towards your end goal!

Except you're not.

In fact, you haven't moved at all.

Here's a riddle for you to explain this concept further:

5 frogs are sitting on a log. 4 frogs decide to jump off. How many frogs are left sitting on the log?

Patiently Waiting For Your Answer.....

Yes! The answer is 5! Great job!

See, 4 of those frogs *decided* to jump off the log. None of them actually jumped.

This is willingness.

Now, I realize I'm not exactly moving mountains with all the inspiring examples I've been giving you but it's not all doom and gloom here.

I just needed you to understand how all of this can either help you or hurt you in your pursuit of change.

When you're in willingness, that means you're opening up yourself to opportunities and possibilities you would have never had if you were stuck in your old, limiting mindset.

Willingness brings freedom of choice.

The choice to climb into the driver seat, buckle in, take the wheel, and forge your own path forward.

Willingness is when you begin to step foot into a new identity and start building your life accordingly.

Willingness sets the stage for our third and final stage of change, which is very specific in what it asks of you:

3. MASSIVE AND CONSISTENT ACTION

Not just massive action.

Not just consistent action.

Both.

Here's why:

If you take massive action one time, you might see a result. But the result would be fleeting and you'd be left with the feeling of, "Wait, that's it?"

If you take small, consistent actions, you will see change. But the time in which it will take you to see progress will most likely open the door for you to get frustrated and disillusioned with the results, so you give up.

You'll see this a lot with New Year's Resolutions.

People set a goal that starting on January 2nd - not January 1st because that's crazy talk - they're going to start making some changes in their lives!

They join a gym, buy a bunch of organic food, pick up a new hobby, stick to the plan for two weeks, and then sink back into the same life they were living the year previously.

If this sounds like you, it's completely ok. You're meant to be here right now. You need to understand this so you can break free from the cycle and start *actually* changing your life.

So, what's the key to taking massive and consistent action?

First, identify what "massive" and "consistent" means to you as it relates to your goal.

For some, it's making 2 new contacts per day in their business. For others, it's going on a date with their significant other every other week.

The qualifications are completely up to you but make sure that, if followed, they would produce noticeable progress towards your end goal in a month's time.

Second, create a non-negotiable rule as it relates to your actions.

Life is bound to throw you some curveballs at some point - this is *expected*. Trying to avoid this would be a futile attempt at pulling a fast one on the universe.

Instead, create a non-negotiable rule that, even in the most dire of circumstances, will ensure that you stay consistent in your pursuit of change.

An example of a non-negotiable rule is if you're trying to get in better shape, you work out three times per week. No exceptions. This means you workout at home, in a gym, in a parking lot, laundry room, Disneyworld, wherever.

It is not up for negotiation whether or not you get that 3rd workout in during the week. You find a way.

What is a non-negotiable rule you will carry forward in your pursuit of change?

_____

After a while, it will just become a part of your daily life.

Speaking of daily life, let's take a look into yours...

CHAPTER TWO

Comfortably
Uncomfortable

"The comfort zone is a psychological state in which one feels familiar, safe, at ease, and secure. You never change your life until you step out of your comfort zone; change begins at the end of your comfort zone."

-Roy T. Bennett

Life will consistently demand more from you than you are willing to give. This is where the entire concept of "comfort zones" came from.

The more demands life places on us, the more pressure we feel to meet those demands. If we don't feel like we can meet the demands of life, we run from them into our comfort zones.

Think of it like being in a sauna.

As the temperature rises, you begin to get a bit uncomfortable, but you can tolerate it. If the temperature gets too high, you'll leave the sauna.

Now, comfort isn't inherently a bad thing. Sometimes comfort is exactly what we need! Life would be miserable if we were always grinding away with no chance to fill back up.

Comfort can also be like drinking alcohol: Enjoyable at first, but too much can ruin your life.

So how do we know when comfort becomes a problem? How much comfort is *too* much comfort?

Let's use an example.

Take Kevin (he's imaginary). Kevin works as an accountant pulling a typical 9-5 weekly work schedule totaling 40 hours every week. This routine rarely ever changes and he loves what he does. After work, Kevin hits the gym for 30 minutes and heads home to make himself dinner. At night during the week, Kevin likes to watch some TV and scroll on his phone. On the weekends, Kevin will occasionally go out to dinner with some of his friends or go for a hike at his favorite trail.

Kevin is very comfortable in his life. He's healthy, he sleeps well, and he feels content. Most importantly, **Kevin is happy.**

Now, let's use the same example character with some different circumstances.

Kevin works as an accountant pulling a typical 9-5 weekly work schedule totaling to 40 hours every week. This routine rarely ever changes and he dreads getting up for work every morning. After work, Kevin goes to a convenience store for a snack; he's not hungry, he just wants to change the way he feels. At night during the week, Kevin distracts himself with some TV and scrolls on his phone to put off going to sleep so he doesn't have to wake up to repeat the same miserable day. On the weekends, Kevin feels so mentally exhausted from his week that he avoids answering his friends when they text him to go out at night. Kevin knows he needs to exercise, but he just can't find the motivation.

Kevin is very comfortable in his life. He's unhealthy, he barely sleeps ,and he feels doomed. Most importantly, **Kevin is unhappy.**

So, how is this possible? How can someone be very comfortable and happy vs. very comfortable and unhappy?

The difference lies in the form of comfort.

Most of us feel stuck in life not because we don't have opportunities; we feel stuck because the opportunities would force us to leave our comfort zone.

We've conditioned ourselves to become comfortably uncomfortable.

In the second example above, Kevin has every opportunity to change his life.

He could quit his soul-sucking job, spend quality time with his friends and take back control of his physique. But all of those things would make him *extremely* uncomfortable.

He'd have to learn new skills. He would have to take bigger risks. He would have to sacrifice some of his TV time and favorite snacks. He would have to suck at something.

When faced with a decision we will always choose the one that inflicts less *perceived* pain. It's our built-in survival mechanism.

We were programmed to avoid pain and seek pleasure. And when life starts demanding more from you, you feel a very strong urge to avoid the pain.

There's an insidious trap inside the state of being comfortably uncomfortable. A trap so deceptive that it should be on every single human being's radar daily.

Ignorance.

See, the problem with becoming comfortably uncomfortable is that you don't realize it's happening until it's too late and you're already deep inside the trap!

Here's a scenario:

A new job takes over your life for 6 months and you let up on your diet and self-care because you're so busy with work. You know you can get back to that *health* stuff any time you want but work is your main priority.

Days go by on what feels like autopilot and you start to lose track of them. One day you wake up, look at your reflection in the mirror and you can't believe what you see. You don't even recognize the person staring back at you. You feel hopeless.

It felt like just yesterday you were loving your life and yourself. But, in reality, you've been creating this for the past 6 months.

That's the trap of being comfortably uncomfortable.

Now some of you might be nodding your head thinking "Hey, that's me!" My heart goes out to you. I know exactly what it feels like and it's a tough situation to find yourself in. But there *is* a way out.

The first step is a difficult one. You have to come to complete acceptance of the fact that you are stuck in this seemingly endless loop.

It sounds easy, but here's what's going to happen:

Your brain is going to start to bargain with you; You'll begin to negotiate.

"It's not that bad."

"It could be worse."

"Tomorrow I'm going to make a change."

"This is the last time."

As many of you reading this most likely know, these statements are rarely true and they lend themselves to an even bigger problem.

When you run an internal dialogue such as the examples listed above, your brain has to make a connection. When the brain makes a connection to an outcome, it prepares itself for that outcome.

Seems reasonable, right?

But what happens when your brain prepares you for a specific outcome that never happens?

And, to take it further, what if your brain keeps preparing you for the same outcome but the outcome consistently doesn't happen? (shoutout to all my over-thinkers)

The answer is you start to lose trust in yourself. You start to realize that you're lying to yourself to pacify the pain of the current moment.

You're justifying being comfortably uncomfortable in your life so you can delay changing.

If you know you need to start losing weight but you find yourself eating chips on the couch in the hour you've set aside to go to the gym and you tell yourself "I'll go tomorrow", you're pacifying the pain of reality.

We'll talk about why this happens later on in the book but I wanted you to get a sneak peek into how our brains will try to sabotage us when we want to make a change.

And before you get ahead of me, the solution to breaking free from being comfortably uncomfortable is not as simple as "get out of your comfort zone."

That may look good as an inspirational quote on Instagram, but it has very little real-world carryover.

How many inspirational quotes have you read that made you think "yeah, that's what I need to do" and then never did anything?

What you need to understand is that getting out of being comfortably uncomfortable takes *time*.

Think about it...

You didn't get into this situation in just a few days.

This was weeks and weeks (for some, years and years) of conditioning your mind, body, spirit, and environment to create the life you feel stuck in.

It's impossible to think that all of this can change overnight - even though that's what the gurus and "woke" people want to sell you.

The truth is that if you want to get out of being comfortably uncomfortable you have to work at it.

Every. Single. Day.

But before you throw this book down and start shaming your comfort zone, there is a process to doing this correctly.

Too much change all at once will actually force you even **deeper** into being comfortably uncomfortable!

I like to call this the "Oh Shit" zone.

If you try changing everything around you at the same time you will create chaos in your mind; It hasn't had the opportunity to adapt to the change, so it won't know how to process the stress associated with making change.

It's pure overwhelm.

This is why most people fail at achieving their goals; They try to change major elements in their life without doing any prep work.

You first stick to **one** thing you want to change (you identified what this change is in the previous chapter).

That's it. Just stick to one. If you try doing more than one you'll get overwhelmed and ultimately fall off track.

Yes, this is me telling you no multitasking.

Get good at one thing outside of your comfort zone before moving onto something else. This is meant to establish a "new" comfort zone.

Once you've decided on what you want to change first, determine what your next step must be to make it a reality.

Is it education? Exercise? Coaching? Mentorship? Investing?

Whatever it is, choose it and ignore the rest. You can get to those after you make progress with this one.

Now, to move forward in this direction of change without giving up early, you can't go for the killshot on the first day.

Change takes time. The length of that time is up to you.

But in order to continually see progress, no matter how long you want it to take, you must employ the principle of One Percent (one of the 4 core change principles we'll talk about later).

By this point, some of you may already be getting uncomfortable by just reading this - that's good! It means this is stirring something in you that's calling you to change.

No one changes until they're ready to put in the work of changing. If you want to change, then you have to commit to change (I'll teach you how in a few chapters).

CHAPTER THREE

Audit Your Life

"Going inward. That's the real work. The solutions are not outside of us. Get to know who you really are, because as you search for the hero within, you inevitably become one."

-Emma Tiebens

When was the last time you really laid out everything you needed to work on in order to get past the point of unfulfillment you're in right now?

I don't just mean thinking about some things you'd like to change; I mean doing a complete life audit to figure out what's working and what's not.

Most of you reading this have never done so and it's a reason you're stuck where you are.

A life audit, put simply, is the sum of everything going on in your life - positive and negative - broken down into individual focus points.

The purpose of the life audit is to bring into full view what you have been avoiding that's currently holding you back, as well as show you everything that's currently working really well for you.

In all elements of change, there is something we tend to avoid. Whether it's a fear, an uncertainty, or an "uncomfortability", we will shy away from that which brings us a sense of "what if this doesn't end well?"

However, it is usually that which we avoid that we must confront first if we plan on making a real change in our lives.

Consider your life as it is right now, and be brutally honest.

What have you been doing well so far? Are you further along than you expected? Less?

In either scenario, there is likely something you have been avoiding. You know what this something is subconsciously, but you have to look at it head on if you want to change it.

I know, this can be uncomfortable. But getting uncomfortable (as we talked about in the previous chapter) is the only way we create lasting change in our lives.

So take a minute now and write down one or two things that you've been avoiding that could change the game for you if you addressed them.

1._____

2._____

After you've identified what you're avoiding, you must look past it.

This doesn't mean ignore it. This means you look into your future and see what your life looks like if you were to address and overcome the things you've been avoiding. The reason for doing this is that you allow yourself to see the possibilities that lie beyond your fear.

Finally, you must put the pieces together and use them to form your strategy for change.

Think of your life like a puzzle. The pieces to your best life will fit if you put them in the right places. But if you don't know where to put the pieces, your life will always feel scattered.

You can overcome anything that comes your way, but it will be much easier if you have an effective plan.

So to start curating this effective plan, we're going to first start with the life audit.

Take out a piece of paper, write below, or take some notes in your phone. If you just read this and try to do it in your head it's going to be significantly less effective and you'll probably forget by the next chapter.

To start the audit, list out every positive thing going on in your life at this moment. When you're done, list every negative.

Everything Positive In My Life:

_____

_____

_____

_____

_____

_____

_____

Everything Negative In My Life:

_____

_____

_____

_____

_____

_____

_____

This exercise is meant to help you start taking everything from thought and place it into reality. You can't escape this and, to some, this sucks (more painful awareness, yay!).

If you find that you have way more negatives than positives, this is called **drowning**.

If you find a close number of positive to negatives, this is called **flatline**.

If you find many more positives than negatives, this is called **growing**.

So, what do these mean to you?

DROWNING

If you're drowning, you're most likely viewing the world through an extremely negative lens.

Everything around you seems to bring you down or remind you of something negative. You find the bad in every good, you focus on what's wrong instead of what's right, and you live in a reserved state of anxious caution waiting to defend yourself against anyone or anything that's "out to get you."

You've found a home in all the negativity you're experiencing daily.

You're trudging through the same problems you've had for the past few years, you battle daily lethargy while rarely ever feeling excited, and creating better habits only lasts for a few days or weeks.

For those of you in this stage...

This is *fucking exhausting*.

The worst part about drowning is we've conditioned ourselves so often to live this way that it's become an automatic response from our nervous system. We've literally programmed our mind to look for negativity and our body to respond accordingly. As a result, we emit an energy that's like a magnet to negativity.

Let me put it another way...

Have you ever been in a room with a bunch of people that are happy and having a good conversation, then all of a sudden somebody comes in and the entire mood changes?

Everyone turns to look at them, the smiles fade, the energy shifts, the conversations stop and the room goes quiet.

This person didn't say or do anything. All they did was walk in the door.

So what happened?

Negative energy.

And the more negative energy you put out, the more you are going to receive in return. This negative energy transfer grows and grows until we start to believe that there is no possibility of finding hope. We believe everyone is out to get us at all times. This is when we start making generalizations and living with all-or-nothing mindsets.

"It's *always* going to be like this."

"They're *never* going to change."

"I'm just *meant to be* alone."

"No one *ever* listens to me."

"This is the *only* way."

By framing your world with absolutes you leave no room for possibility. And when there's no room for possibility, you sink deeper into negativity.

That's why it's called drowning.

FLATLINE

Believe it or not, being in flatline is actually worse than drowning.

Flatline tricks you into thinking everything is ok until you wake up ten years later and realize it's absolutely not. Cue mid-life crisis.

Imagine driving 2500 continuous miles in your car. For reference, that's a little less than the width of the United States.

You were headed out from the East Coast to visit a friend in California.

During the entire drive, the temperature inside the car keeps shifting from uncomfortably warm, to comfortable, to uncomfortably cold every 10 minutes. And you never know when it's going to change within that 10 minute timeframe.

It's total chaos fueled by uncertainty. As soon as you start to feel like the temperature is where you want it to be and your body gets used to it, it starts to creep towards being uncomfortable.

It's annoying. It's unpredictable. It's confusing. Like life!

But you can deal with it because *sometimes* it feels ok. And when it feels ok, the drive is enjoyable.

Now imagine you've reached what you thought was the end of your trip, the 2500 miles to see your friend, and you can't wait to be done with this miserable car ride.

You get out of the car, stiff and irritated, and walk into a local shop to see if they can point you in the right direction. When you approach the shop owner, you tell them which town your friend lives in and you're wondering if you're in the right spot.

The shop owner shakes his head and says, "It's about 75 more miles from here."

Now you have to choose whether or not to get back into your temperature nightmare of a car and complete the trip or you can address the issue and stop the torture. You have no idea how long fixing the car is going to take, or how expensive it might be, or if you can even find anyone to fix it. But you *do* know you can handle that car's temperature being miserable just a little longer because for a few minutes here and there, it doesn't feel too bad.

This is flatlining.

This pattern appears most in people who aren't where they want to be but they're not where they were. Their life is "OK." They have a stable job, livable salary, a couple friends, maybe a family.

But they feel passionless. They feel like there is so much more they could do. They feel limited in their life or held back. They want to grow but they don't want to lose what they have. They're trapped in a "damned if I do, damned if I don't" mentality. It's a constant push and pull of feeling guilty for wanting to better themselves while simultaneously feeling guilty for *not* bettering themselves.

Flatliners are often very anxious and have wavering confidence in themselves.

Flatlining is a dangerous pattern because the further you get away from it, the harder it tries to pull you back in. **It's a pattern of relief.** And since we can't always be grinding and burning ourselves out, sometimes we really want that relief.

But relief takes your foot off the gas. You don't press the brake and you don't accelerate. You just....coast.

And then one day you wake up and realize you've been coasting for the last 20 years. This is when panic ensues. This is when we question ourselves intensely. This is when we feel the full pain of regret of not going after the things we really want.

GROWING

Growing is obviously the most beneficial place to be. Growing is defined by positivity.

Those of you in the growing stage probably have a very optimistic outlook on the world. A problem is never a problem, just something you have to address. People are here to help you, not hurt you. Your potential is limitless as long as you put in the work.

Before I explain this concept any further I want to make something completely clear:

Growing IS NOT just thinking positively. Positive *thinking* without positive *action* is useless.

If you had a horrible allergic reaction to something you ate, just thinking positively that it will go away could *literally* kill you. You have to address the reaction, take action to prevent yourself from injury or death, *and then* think positively about the outcome.

Growing means seeking out the good in life and looking for ways to continue growing as a human being.

Inherently, we all desire growth. If we don't grow, we die - spiritually, emotionally, and sometimes physically.

Those of you that are growing are probably often misunderstood, looked upon as fake; classified as "ignorant", "selfish", "cocky", or "arrogant". You're dealing with those in a fixed mindset while you live in a growth-based mindset. These two mindsets don't get along.

Coincidentally, those in the growing category of life also tend to have more opportunities. They have better life circumstances. They get better jobs. They make more money. They're often much happier.

This, once again, goes directly back to energy. What they are putting out is exactly what they are getting back.

So what does this look like in action?

People that are growing are often only understood by others that are also growing. To everyone else, growing looks like someone is dismissive of problems or showing off. Sometimes it can appear as though people that are growing are not sympathetic or think only about themselves and can't relate to other people.

In reality, those that are growing know the value of positive energy and surrounding themselves with people that contribute to that energy is one of their top priorities. If too much negative energy is brought upon them, someone in the growing category could be dragged down to flatlining or drowning very quickly.

A QUICK NOTE ON PEOPLE AND PLACES IN YOUR LIFE

Most of you reading this probably have the same immediate social and professional circles that you've had for years. How many of those in your immediate circle would you want to trade places with?

Who you spend time with is almost crucial to your entire success in the end. Can you guess why?

Because they have the most influence on your life.

There's a common saying that goes, "If you hang out with 4 losers, you'll be the 5th."

Think about it. The 5 people that you spend the most time *with* are also probably the 5 people you would do the most *for*.

Sometimes "doing something for them" turns into doing *everything* for them.

Ever feel like you're the only one giving, yet you're so unfulfilled yourself?

Before you put the rest of your life into the hands of your coworkers, friends, and loved ones, I need you to think about yourself.

Make a list of all the people you know, and pick out the best 5 that would *truly stand by you and support you* throughout your entire journey of change.

Are those five that would support you in your every day circle? All of them? Some? None?

Figure out who the best influences to your life are, and incorporate ways to see them or talk with them more often. They will be your best support system as you change.

Trying to change your life alone is one of the worst strategies ever conceived on this planet.

The five people you spend the most time with are ALMOST all of the equation.

In order to truly take control of your future, you'll have to also analyze the 5 places you spend the most time *in*. Usually, you will find that the 5 people you spend the most time with have a high correlation to where you spend most of your time.

Are those environments conducive to your success? Will they allow you the tools needed to do what you need to do or be who you need to be?

What are some better environments you could be in to help you as you progress?

Simply putting yourself in a new, empowering environment will open your world up to so many new experiences, opportunities, and connections.

So now what?

Now is the time to look inward and take a true evaluation of where you believe yourself to be in this current moment in time. Are you drowning, flatlining, or growing?

The principles in this book are going to teach you how to move up the scale, so don't be too discouraged if you realize you're somewhere you don't want to be. This is just a starting point of your journey.

CHAPTER FOUR

The Only 3 Things Keeping You From Change

*"There are very few monsters
who warrant the fear we have
of them"*

-Andre Gide

In the next chapter, we're going to dive into the core life change principles of the book. But before we get there, we need to lay some groundwork.

Some of you reading this are totally engaged right now.

You're clinging to every word, you're associating with the concepts, you're taking notes, and you're actively applying the information you're learning to your life.

That's excellent. Keep doing that.

Now, on the other hand, some of you are just passively reading this.

Maybe you've read a little bit here and there and have put the book down multiple times to get distracted by useless material. You've spaced the chapters out for weeks because you don't like reading. Whatever your reasons are, they're there.

I get it. I've been there too.

Which is why we're going to address the most important equation of your life:

Focus + Action = Outcome

How many of you have already lost focus while reading this book?

Better question, how many of you have checked your phone—or are currently looking at your phone—as you're reading this?

If this is you, then I know that I don't have your full attention.

Hard to believe since this book is, you know, *incredible*.

If I don't have your attention, then I definitely don't have your focus. And your focus is needed for any of this to work.

So pay attention.

Your mind will assist you, or resist you, depending on where your focus is.

If you focus on your lack of confidence or belief in your abilities, chances are your mind will be working against you.

If you focus on your destination, and what you want to accomplish, consistently and accurately, your mind will dial itself into the goal. This is the trick that separates successful people from people that consistently fail.

It's not about talent or resources. It's not about confidence or opportunities. And it's most certainly not about luck.

Those are all variables.

The one universal, concrete skill that will help bring you success is the ability to control your focus and zero in on what you *want* instead of what you *don't want*.

Most of us have a hard time with this if we are constantly surrounded by things that distract us or cause us to focus on negativity. Interestingly enough, what you focus on could actually keep you stuck longer than you would believe.

Consider someone that is, or has been, depressed. Odds are, they do not have very encouraging thoughts. But why is this? Is nothing good happening in their life? They might say so, but the reason this happens is simple.

When we find ourselves in an unresourceful state (anxious, scared, sad, depressed), our minds tend to gravitate towards thoughts that will satisfy the emotion we are experiencing - this a major reason why people have a hard time letting go of the past.

If something painful happened to them in the past that made them strongly associate with a negative emotion - say divorce and loneliness - then every time they feel lonely, their mind will give them the opportunity to call back on the painful memories of the divorce. Then focus takes over and makes the situation infinitely worse.

We can find ways to amplify the strength of our emotions by focusing on the right things at the right times. The more intensely you focus on something, the more it consumes you.

So, if you focus on how to stay happy while you're already happy, you'll find ways to do so. Likewise, you can find ways to get more angry when you are already experiencing anger.

The challenge is to pull yourself out of a negative emotion and into a positive one utilizing only your focus. And the more you do this, the easier it will become.

I won't beg you to read this or take what I'm saying to heart. But I will tell you that the remaining chapters of this book, including this one, will absolutely change your life...

IF YOU PAY ATTENTION AND USE THE INFORMATION.

Because if you don't you'll stay stuck in the same patterns, you'll encounter the same problems, and you'll continue living unfulfilled for far longer than you expect.

With that said, let's talk about what's really keeping you from changing.

DOUBT, FEAR, AND HESITATION

We're creatures of desire.

In fact, that's why you're even reading this: you desire change.

The desires we have are rarely un-attainable, yet we find ways to talk ourselves out of getting what we want because we don't see it as possible.

Ultimately, we start to develop a weak sense of self-worth if we're not on track to getting what we want.

Take a moment right now and think of something significant you've wanted to have in your life.

This desire could be materialistic, like a nice house or a dream car. It could be born of love, such as having a passionate relationship or a beautiful family. Or it could be a product of your own doing, such as starting your own business.

I want you to imagine what it is that you truly desire and spend a minute or two immersing yourself in that vision. If you already have many of the things you want in life, focus on how you can have even more or improve upon them.

Now, as you were visualizing what you wanted, did it seem more like a dream or a reality? Did it feel like you were destined to attain this or that "it would be nice to have?"

If it felt more like a dream than reality, your belief system is preventing you from achieving that desire.

Lucky for you, changing our beliefs is one of the simplest things we can do to enhance our lives. But please don't think I'm telling you it's easy. Simple and easy are two totally separate concepts.

Over the course of my career, I've picked up on a few key patterns that keep people from getting what they want; especially when it comes to a goal or desire.

If I told you that by changing only 3 beliefs you could have anything you want, would you be willing to pay me for it? What if I then proceeded to tell you what those 3 beliefs were and how to reframe them to serve your needs, what about then?

I'm in a good mood, so I'll make you a deal. I'll teach you what 3 beliefs are keeping you from getting what you want and how to reframe them for the low, low price of.....

Absolutely nothing!

(or, technically, the amount of money you already paid for this book).

I *will* request a different form of payment. If you read these strategies, you must make a dedicated attempt to implement them into your life to create positive change.

Remember, knowledge is not power. The *application* of knowledge is power.

AKA stop thinking and start doing.

Without further ado, I give you:

The ONLY Three Things Keeping You From Change.

1 - DOUBT

What will never cease to amaze me about humankind is our unrelenting ability to lose faith in ourselves. Even worse, we tend to count ourselves out before we even begin.

Doubt will stop you in your tracks, and could result in you getting off the tracks entirely. By letting doubts cloud our vision, we begin to eliminate possibilities. We mentally delete outcomes because we don't believe they're possible to achieve.

Doubt is usually the result of a lack of information or certainty.

If we don't know what will happen in the future or we are lacking the necessary information to know positively that what we want is possible, we will begin to doubt our ability to make it happen.

Typically, doubt is the catalyst for inactivity.

You see this a lot in people with limited skill sets or little experience of the world. They're often unsure of themselves and approach much of life with caution. Caution isn't always a bad thing, but too much caution is crippling.

If you find yourself doubting most of the things you do on a daily basis, you're probably struggling to gain any real traction in this life.

Think of doubt like a leech.

It sinks its teeth in you, latches on, and sucks out your self-confidence. And the more often you doubt yourself, the more leeches begin to latch on.

When we doubt ourselves, we are less likely to put forth a concentrated effort towards getting what we want. If we doubt long enough, we encounter our second element of dream robbing:

2 - FEAR

Fear sucks.

It always finds its way around in some form or fashion, produces anxiety, and can control almost all of our focus.

But do you know why fear really sucks? Because it's not real.

We create it.

And the more fear we create, the stronger it becomes.

Fear is a product of what I like to call the "what if" factor.

- What if my business fails and I go broke?
- What if my significant other leaves me?
- What if I get what I want and I'm not happy?
- What if it's not really what I want?
- What if, what if, what if.....

We tend to assume the worst-case scenario will always play out, and that the best-case scenario isn't possible.

Yet both scenarios are equal in reality if you have not yet attempted going after what you want.

We're primed to think in worst case scenarios because our nervous system is actively alert for threats. We're wired for defense.

Think of primal human beings.

We needed to survive in our early, knuckle-dragging days. In order to survive, we had to be on the lookout for threats and things that could kill us. Harsh conditions, predatory animals, famine, thirst, shelter, disease; the list is endless.

As a result of this concern for our well-being, our minds evolved to automatically seek out danger with the purpose of protecting ourselves from it.

Now, with the exception of a few populations, we don't need to be on high alert for predators and harsh living conditions constantly, yet our brains continue looking for it.

This is why fear can be so prevalent: **protection.**

Ultimately your fears are really there to protect you, but most fear is irrational. We very often fear things that never happen or don't exist.

Remember this: fear is not real, danger is.

Fear is designed to alert us of danger, but fear cannot do anything more than trigger alertness. Danger can absolutely hurt you depending on what the danger actually is.

If a stranger is walking up to you and you feel fear of being attacked, you're being put on alert. However, you have no idea what the stranger wants. They could be asking you for directions for all you know up to this point. The fear has no substance, just imagination fueled by uncertainty of what this person wants.

Now, if a stranger is walking up to you with a knife in their hand and threatens to stab you....yeah, you're in danger. You should be very afraid and use that fear to protect yourself.

But too often we confuse fear and danger.

We also mis-label what it is that we're actually afraid of, creating a false belief of what *actually* scares us.

For example:

- You're not afraid of heights, you're afraid of falling.

- You're not afraid of the dark, you're afraid of what might be in it.
- You're not afraid of sharks, you're afraid of getting attacked by them.

When we fear the outcome of something, we don't take action (or *consistent* action) in the direction of making that thing a reality. We associate pain to the outcome and we do everything in our power to avoid it.

Remember that first time you took the training wheels off your bike as a kid?

Or that first school dance?

Or when you had a crush on someone for what seemed like forever and you finally mustered up the courage to tell them?

Remember that hollow feeling in your gut as you were preparing to do all these?

That's called fear.

Here's why I ask:

In all of those situations you had to overcome the fear of failure, pain, rejection, or disappointment to achieve your goal. You may have hesitated for a while before following through with it, but you eventually did.

And when you did, you learned two things:

1. Failure sucks, but it's really not as bad as it seems in your head
2. You were stronger than your fear

As kids, we learn to overcome fear daily. Sometimes we're forced to, and other times we choose to. This is how we learn and grow.

And we had no choice *but* to grow. We learned everything we needed to learn about ourselves at a young age and we used it daily. Sometimes the fear won, and sometimes we did. But we never stopped trying.

Which brings me to now.

What are you afraid of now?

Because we get to a point in life where riding a bike without training wheels becomes leaving (or saving) a 15 year relationship that's draining us of our soul.

Getting ready for a school dance becomes starting a business or changing careers completely after having spent most of our life working in one field.

Telling your crush you like them becomes seeking help for your depression that you've been silently battling for the better part of your adult life.

The difference between the younger us and the older us is that when we were younger, we didn't let our fear cripple us for years before we did something about it. We tried and failed forward. The stakes seemed astronomical at the time and we still chose to take on the challenge, not knowing what the outcome was going to be.

The longer you let fear build up, the harder it becomes to face. But every day you hold onto fear is another day clinging to a hidden pain.

Whatever your fear, you *can* overcome it. I promise.

You've had to make extremely tough decisions in the past. Decisions that you probably thought were going to ruin you, crush you, or kill you.

But here you are. Reading a book about changing your life and choosing to grow.

Most people don't make it out of the fear stage and give up prematurely. The determined ones that don't give up when faced with fear arrive at the third element keeping them from change.

3 - HESITATION

Remember when you were young and all of your friends were learning to swim underwater? I know I do.

-If you can't swim underwater, let my story inspire you.
-If you can't swim at all, I *highly* encourage you to learn.

I specifically remember being terrified to put my head under the water for fear of drowning. Even though all of my friends were doing it, I couldn't pull myself to do it. I would do the bare minimum. I would put my chin under, eventually my nose, I would dunk my face but not my whole head; I just couldn't pull myself to go all the way under!

Until one day I decided I was going to do it. I mustered up the courage to get into the pool with the mindset of going underwater. Keep in mind I was like 5, so this was a big moment for me.

When the time came to go under, I froze. I was terrified. All my courage left. Fear was taking over, and I was hesitating.

And I hesitated for about 20 minutes.

Thankfully, a good friend of mine dunked me underwater and I had no chance to hesitate anymore.

Was I mad? Absolutely.

Startled? Yes.

Did I go under again that day? You bet I did.

Moral of the story is that my fear was producing my hesitation, and that hesitation was bringing me nowhere closer to my goal; rather, it was preventing it.

Here's how hesitation sabotages us just before we make a change.

We've already gone through the first initial phase of change prep: doubt. After successfully overcoming our doubts we move into phase 2: fear. After stepping into our fear we have one final move to make; one monumental moment that could change our future...

But we hesitate. We hesitate because we still don't have certainty that we're going to be OK on the other side of change.

And the longer we hesitate, the bigger gap we create for doubt and fear to start winning the fight again.

There is a direct correlation to the amount of time in which we hesitate and how much we believe we can achieve.

If you're someone that often avoids or procrastinates, you've conditioned yourself to do these things before taking action. This is called a pattern.

Action teaches lessons, hesitation strengthens patterns.

Our doubts, fears, and hesitations provide the recipe for limiting our potential and preventing us from getting what we really want.

You're going to learn how to turn these negative mindsets into power in the coming chapters.

CHAPTER FIVE

The Core Principles of Change

"The only way to make sense out of change is to plunge into it, move with it, and join the dance."

-Alan Watts

If you're still with me, this is where the fun begins.

I have no doubts that you've already started growing by reading the previous chapters, but we're throwing gas on the fire from this chapter forward. My goal is to completely open your eyes to new possibilities for you and give you the opportunity to choose to live a better life. And with this book, and the change principles you're about to learn, you'll have all the tools you need to make immediate change.

The Core Principles of Change have been developed over years and years of coaching people to break through their negative mindsets, overcome their limiting circumstances, and reinvent their lives. Most everyone that was successful in changing their life followed The Core Principles of Change. Those that didn't follow the principles typically fell back into their old patterns and habits within weeks of our coaching conclusion.

These core change principles were created to address common problems I was seeing in most of my clients, my social circle and friend groups, my colleagues at work, and even myself.

I wanted to create something simple that could remind myself and others how to pull themselves out of a negative mindset or living situation and start re-inventing the way they lived.

I knew there were a million concepts at play, but complexity is the enemy of progress. So I narrowed it down to only four key principles.

IF you follow all 4 change principles, you will live a better life. *Guaranteed.*

Bold statement, right?

I'd be willing to risk my entire reputation on it.

But before we get any further into it, I have to talk about the importance in having principles such as these.

If you live your life without any sort of direction or standards, like the change principles we're going to talk about in just a moment, you'll typically end up living in whatever way your environment determines for you. You'll make the same decisions, have the same problems, and repeat the same cycles over and over again until you finally realize you need some discipline.

Holding yourself to a higher standard is an almost bulletproof strategy at making changes in your life without needing anything more than you already have inside you.

By raising your standards and demanding more from yourself, you'll start exercising your self-confidence muscle. As this muscle grows, you'll begin to notice your belief in yourself growing as well. This belief strengthening occurs because you're finally taking responsibility for your life and everything that happens within it. You're in the driver's seat.

It's those without discipline or standards that fall victim to their circumstance.

The Core Principles of Change I've created specifically to push you out of your comfort zone and pull you towards the life you want.

These 4 principles have the power to take you from where you are to where you want to be in record time with jaw-dropping efficiency.

They'll unlock skills and talents in you that you never thought existed.

You'll start to have more and more opportunities reveal themselves right before your eyes.

This is the most simple and effective way to change your life.

But a word of caution.....

If you read these principles and don't implement them, you will stay where you are.

If you read these principles and only implement them occasionally, you will stay where you are.

For these 4 principles to work, you must practice them every single day until they become a part of your daily life.

This is extremely simple, but not easy.

I don't say any of this to scare you; Quite the opposite.

I want to inspire you to take some real action and make some real changes in your life!

Too many articles, books, and quotes give you words.

I want to give you change. I want to give you action.

The Core Principles of Change

PRINCIPLE 1: NO ONE IS COMING TO SAVE YOU

PRINCIPLE 2: ONE PERCENT

PRINCIPLE 3: DCA (DECIDE. COMMIT. ACT)

PRINCIPLE 4: PRIORITIZE GROWTH

"NODP" if you want an acronym to remember them by. It doesn't really make sense, but now you have a way of shortening the principles. Plus acronyms are awesome for memory retention.

So you get "NODP."

CHAPTER SIX

Principle 1: No One Is Coming To Save You

"You have brains in your head. You have feet in your shoes. You can steer yourself any direction you choose. You're on your own. And you know what you know. And YOU are the one who'll decide where to go..."

- Dr. Seuss

Most of us spend years of our lives waiting for something to change.

Year after year we break promises to ourselves that we're going to improve our bodies, we're going to be more positive, we're going to try new things, yada yada yada.

After a while, we stop believing in our own abilities to do anything and we just simply wait.

We wait for someone to come along and pull us out of pain.

We wait for the "right" time and the "right" opportunity to fall into our lap.

We wait and hope that one day we're going to wake up to a letter in the mailbox that says, "Congratulations! Here's that change you wanted so badly."

But that day never comes and the letter never arrives. The opportunity doesn't fall into our laps. No one comes to pull us out of pain.

In the depths of our most troubling times, we will cling to the belief that someone—or something—will give us the answers we need to live a better life.

- Some put their faith in religion or family.

- Some turn to friends.

- Some turn to therapists or counselors.

Very few turn to themselves.

The responsibility of changing can be a heavy weight to bear, especially if you don't know how to change or you feel like you've been stuck in a repeating cycle all your life.

You *have* to take complete ownership of your life. The good, the bad, the ugly, and the confusing.

If your life isn't the way you want it to be, it is 100% your responsibility to change it. You must be your own savior.

I can't tell you the amount of people I've talked with or coached that have said the phrases "I've always been like this" or "That's just who I am."

Look, if you want to stay the exact same as you are with the same low-quality problems and limiting mindsets, stop reading this right now.

Committing yourself to a life of "That's just who I am" is a death sentence to who you *could* be.

But there's a reason we default to these absolute identities.

Changing is hard work. And it would be so much easier if we could just rely on someone else to come by and help us change faster.

Don't get me wrong, I will always encourage seeking out help or hiring a coach to assist you in making a change. But most people wait until they've wasted valuable years of their life to take responsibility and start the change process.

And that's where principle number 1 comes into play: **No One is Coming to Save You.**

It is your responsibility and your responsibility alone to make a change in your life. This *does not* mean that you have to know everything required to make the change. Quite the opposite is true. All you have to do is actually make a dedicated effort to the change itself.

By adhering to this principle, you will put the power back in your control. Blaming outside circumstances or other people for the negative things going on in your life will do nothing but strip power from you.

Instead, focus on the fact that no matter what happens from this point on, change starts and ends with you. YOU are the only one that can save you.

This seems simple in theory, but wait until you hit a low point and you want to start pointing fingers.

Wait until the responsibilities start stacking up.

Wait until your insecurities and limiting beliefs take over for a second.

These are the defining moments where you get to make a choice:

I can let my circumstances define me or I can define my circumstances.

If you can adopt this principle, you can find a way to do almost anything.

Say you're faced with a situation where you don't know what to do next.

Instead of taking some form of action, you just wait. You wait for someone to tell you what the next step is. You wait for the right moment. You wait until you feel "ready."

The entire time you're waiting you're also noticing that nothing is actually improving and your situation is just getting worse.

If you adopted the principle that No One is Coming to Save You, you would start from where you are with the resources that you have and you would begin creating your solution because it's the only way forward. No longer will you feel the need to wait for something better to come along.

This principle is designed to make you resourceful.

The more resourceful you become the more opportunities you're going to have in this life. Not because you're going to just stumble upon opportunity; it's because you're going to be the one creating the opportunities.

Being resourceful in your pursuit of change can make your life a whole lot easier. It will also help you grow immensely as a person.

The textbook definition of resourcefulness is "the ability to find quick and clever ways to overcome difficulties."

My definition is "the ability to rely on yourself."

If you want to truly take control of your future, you must rely heavily on your ability to be resourceful. You will find success much easier this way because you are becoming a student of your own life. You are pursuing the answers most prevalent to you, in order to have that information for a future time when the same situation comes up.

If you take nothing else from this program, get more resourceful!

I've found that I solve problems much faster than most of my peers not because I'm any smarter than them, I just pursue the answer more diligently.

Nowadays, you can be resourceful in literal seconds by pulling out your smart phone.

The internet is the best resourcefulness tool of all time.

Think about it, you have access to the world's information at your fingertips. If you're ever stuck in life all you have to do is reach into your pocket, pull out your phone, and search for the answer to your problem.

You'll find chat forums of people that have already overcome the exact struggle you're in right now. You'll find peer reviewed articles defining your exact situation, causes, and solutions. You'll find blogs specializing in helping people that are exactly like you.

You still think you can't find a solution to your struggle on your own? Of course you can; you already have everything you need.

Here's an example of Brenda. She's also imaginary, but pretend she's not.

Brenda has been trying dating websites for a few months but still can't seem to find a relationship. In the midst of an emotional spiral, Brenda decides to do some research.

"I'm feeling sad that I can't get into a relationship. Why do I feel this way? Is it because I'm lonely? Is it because I'm frustrated? I'm not sure. Hang on, I'll check."

Brenda types into the internet search bar: "Why do I feel sad that I can't get into a relationship?"

Millions of results come up.

She sees an article titled "Why You Feel Sad You Aren't In A Relationship."

Brenda clicks it and reads. She resonates very heavily with a section that discusses that "normally you are not feeling sad that you aren't in a relationship, you're feeling sad about your current state in life and you think that a relationship will bring you happiness because you haven't found a way to be happy on your own."

Brenda has been thinking a lot recently about how she isn't happy with her looks and her weight. Her poor image of herself has almost completely crippled her self-confidence. She noticed that she points out all of her insecurities on her dating websites and overthinks everything she puts on there.

Brenda also realized that she no longer takes care of herself. She no longer wears make-up, fancy clothes, or pays attention to her personal hygiene.

In this moment, Brenda realizes that she must be able to love herself if she expects to love anyone else.

Brenda sets out on a new course of action and focuses completely on herself. She starts working out, improves her mental health, tries new makeup, and buys some new clothes.

After a few months, Brenda loves the direction her life is heading in. She feels great, she looks great, and she's beginning to really love herself.

She's starting to go back out into social environments, makes plans with friends, tries new hobbies, and expands her social circle.

She catches the attention of a guy one day. He sees how happy and free she seems to be, which is something he desires in his perfect match. He goes up to Brenda to introduce himself, they hit it off, and a few weeks later......BOOM! Relationship.

All because of a quick internet search Brenda made one day.

This is the true power of resourcefulness.

* * *

HEAVY LIES THE CROWN

In the deepest, darkest pits of your journey through life, you will face tremendous adversity.

Not from your friends or families. Not from enemies. But from yourself.

You will feel beaten and bruised.

You will lose all hope and motivation.

You will feel that you are wasting away into a "is this really all there is?" existence.

And your brain will stop looking for solutions to pull you out of pain.

This is the defining moment of your life.

If you don't want to take on the responsibility of changing your life, then you will live out your days feeling how you feel now.

If, however, you rise up and embrace the gift of opportunity you have before you right now, you will grow and thrive in ways you haven't yet imagined.

I know this may seem impossible for some of you but I beg you, stay open-minded.

If you've never accomplished anything that's made you proud or you still feel like you're not good enough then make this point right now, today, your starting line in a marathon of self-improvement.

You don't have to be great right now.

You don't even have to be good right now.

In fact, it's ok to be in the worst place you've ever been right now!

But it's not ok to stay there.

If you accept the responsibility of changing your life, you have an actual shot at changing it.

CHAPTER SEVEN

Principle 2: One Percent

"The only way that we can live, is if we grow. The only way that we can grow is if we change. The only way that we can change is if we learn. The only way we can learn is if we are exposed. And the only way that we can become exposed is if we throw ourselves out into the open. Do it. Throw yourself."

- C. JoyBell C.

If you've been down on your luck for a while now, you probably think change is impossible.

You probably feel doomed to repeat the same monotonous day over and over again until you eventually die from something you could have prevented had you only made some lifestyle changes.

Or you spend most of your days stuck inside your own head, desperately hoping for that one day where your confidence skyrockets and you start living the life you know you deserve.

There's only one problem with both of these...

YOU'RE NOT DOING ANYTHING.

Sorry, let me rephrase.

You're not doing enough of the *right* things.

And I'm not going to tell you what the right things are because you already know what they are. Instinctively, you know. That's why you're not doing them. They scare you.

It would be unethical for me to sell you answers you already have. It's my job to pull them out of you.

- If you're overweight, you already know you need to start eating better and taking your physical health more seriously.

- If you're depressed, you know you need to spend more time being active, challenging yourself, changing your internal self-talk, creating new beliefs about what's possible for your life, and growing as a human being.

- If you're broke, you know you need to start putting yourself out there more and grinding a little bit harder to start making some money.

But you *already* know this! And that's why the principle of One Percent is so effective.

The principle of One Percent states that each day, you strive to be one percent better than you were the day before. Whatever one percent is to you is completely your decision, but it should not be something that is so emotionally or physically demanding of you that it's not sustainable.

Remember, we're looking for consistent, long term growth here. The main reason so many people fail when they're trying to make a change is that they overwhelm themselves with way too much, too fast.

So here's how the principle of One Percent works.

I don't want you to spend all your time thinking of the end goal (although, I want it to stay in your vision), I don't want you to hyper focus on whether or not you're doing the right things, and I definitely don't want you trying to rush this change.

Your mission, from this point forward, is to **be one percent closer to your goal EVERY. SINGLE. DAY.**

Now, let's really think about this in application.

If you improved by one percent every day from the start of this chapter to the end of 30 days, how much further along in your life do you believe you would be?.

And for those of you thinking, "...but you told us taking small, consistent actions won't help us be successful in chapter 1." Hear me out.

If you grow by one percent from where you are right now every single day, you could be completely separated from the negativity and self-limitations you're living in long enough to start making some serious momentum for change. One percent growth each day may not seem like a lot, but you have to remember...this isn't a quick fix. And this principle is empowering you to take bigger actions each day, rather than simply repeating the same actions over and over until you get bored and stop trying.

If you were to implement the principle of One Percent for an entire year, all of your progress would begin compounding on itself and growing exponentially - all from making small improvements every day.

One percent growth each day is MASSIVE, life altering change when viewed on a year timeline.

This entire book is designed to set you up for long term success and give you the tools necessary to reinvent your life, but this principle alone will take you places you never thought possible if followed properly.

And the beauty of the principle of One Percent is *now* you have the ability to utilize this method for everything else in your life that needs it. I have found that the principle of One Percent not only helps people change, but helps them maintain that change for good.

So, now it's your turn to get real with yourself. What can you start doing right now, one percent better than yesterday, to move in the direction of your best life?

I'll give you an example if you need a jumpstart.

Say you wanted to lose some weight but you had no idea where to begin, so you looked up a fitness article on fat loss diets. Then the next day, in honor of One Percent, you read two articles. Then, on day 3, you made a recipe that you found in those articles. On day 4, you tried one of the exercise routines you saw in an email your friend sent you. So on and so forth.

Will this formula change you overnight? No. But it will prime you for continued success since you are building off of knowledge and implementing what you're learning into your life in a sustainable way.

In time, looking up fitness articles and trying new recipes/workouts will become a part of your "new" comfort zone.

I started my career as a personal trainer (hence why you'll hear me reference a lot of fitness stories and weight loss related examples).

The principle of One Percent was created because I saw how discouraged people would get when they wanted to make massive changes in their lives, but felt completely overwhelmed with how long they believed it was going to take them.

And in a world where everyone is trying to sell you a quick fix, this often led many people to trying fad diets or programs that didn't work for them - resulting in frustration, beliefs that they couldn't change, and wasted time/money/energy.

Once they started implementing the principle of One Percent, they were excited about changing because they *knew* they were making progress every day, even if just a small amount.

It also helped with holding themselves accountable when they were having a bad day or didn't feel like working on themselves.

And I understand that not everyone is after any goal fitness related, so let me give you another example.

I was coaching a man who wanted to develop a deeper relationship with his then girlfriend. For privacy, we'll call him Steve.

Steve and his girlfriend had been together for a few years and he was feeling as though they were drifting apart. They barely connected with each other, all intimacy had stopped, and it felt tense to simply be in each other's presence. Steve knew he wanted to fix things between him and his woman, but he didn't know how to bring the two of them back together.

After a few coaching sessions, Steve realized that he had been very focused on himself and his career for a full 6 months. He rarely ever checked in with his girlfriend to see how it was impacting her or if there were anything he could be doing better as a partner.

Steve felt embarrassed, overwhelmed, and defeated.

"This is a perfect opportunity for you to utilize the principle of One Percent," I told him, then explaining what the principle entailed.

Steve initially laughed because he didn't think it would be enough to salvage what they had. Still, I encouraged him to give a full-out effort for the next 30 days at growing their relationship by one percent each day. He agreed.

In our follow up session two weeks later, I asked him for an update on how things were going between him and his girlfriend.

Steve burst out with excitement and told me everything he had been doing for her and how he was growing the relationship by one percent each day.

- The first day, he told her she looked nice as she was leaving for work.

- The next day, he sat with her while she watched her favorite show.

- The day after, he wrote her a little love note and put it in her lunch bag so she could find it at work and think of him.

- After a week, they were spending twice the amount of time together as they had previously.

- Within two weeks, they had been on 2 dates, they were texting each other all day long, and they were intimate again.

At the time of writing this, they're engaged to be married. Steve told me that they continue to try growing their relationship by one percent every day to further deepen their love and passion for each other.

Did this take Steve an absurd amount of time and effort to rekindle a dying flame with his soon-to-be wife?

Absolutely not. Each little act of effort took less than an hour, some as little as two minutes. But the results speak for themselves.

* * *

QUICK DISCLAIMER

Talking about the principle of one percent is one thing. Determining how you want to grow by one percent is a step in the right direction. But nothing will happen if you don't take action. Which brings us to...

CHAPTER EIGHT

Principle 3: D.C.A
(Decide. Commit. Act.)

"None of it works unless YOU work. We have to do our part. If knowing is half the battle, action is the second half of the battle."
- Jim Kwik

DECIDE

How many decisions do you think you make every single day?

- When to wake up
- When to eat
- What to eat
- When to sleep
- How much work to do
- Who to talk to
- Who to avoid
- What to think about
- Etc.

The list can go on and on, filled with decisions.

But what happens when we have to make the tough decisions? What happens when we have to make decisions that scare us? What happens when we have to make decisions that could involve failure, loss of love, loss of finances, loss of our identity, etc.

Most of us decide to do nothing - which is the worst decision we can make. And yes, that's still a decision.

To take it further, many of us decide to do nothing, *even when we know what we have to do.*

When we decide to do nothing, after knowing what we have to do, we start to lose trust in ourselves to do the right thing. And as we make more of these decisions to do nothing, the worse we begin to feel.

This is when the word "should" starts to enter our daily vocabulary.

We tell ourselves (and everyone else) that we *should* do something other than what we're doing.

- I should call my dad
- I should workout
- I should eat better
- I should watch less tv
- I should give more of an effort at work
- I should read more
- I should meditate
- I should go to the doctor
- I should get a hobby

Soon enough, "should" becomes our favorite word. And when we start to feel bad enough about our decision to do nothing, we decide to distract ourselves so we don't have to make any decisions at all (again, that's still a decision).

Why?

Because decisions can be painful. And we will do whatever we can to avoid pain.

Ok, so, back to you and your decisions...

Making decisions can be very similar to positive thinking; just because you made a decision doesn't change anything about your current situation. But we find ways to trick ourselves into believing that because we've finally decided to make a change, we've accomplished something (remember our frogs on the log from earlier?).

A decision without action is a deception.

Think about it this way:

If you were going to go skydiving, you would have to first decide that you are indeed going to go skydiving.

Your next decision would be that you are going to get into a plane and put a parachute on.

The next decision you would make is that once the time is right, you will jump out of that plane.

Pretty straightforward, right?

Well all of this decision making can make you feel very resolute and confident in your ability to skydive. You might even feel like you've accomplished something big by just making this decision.

But in order to skydive, *you have to fucking skydive.*

Don't fall victim to the illusion that by just making a decision you are going to experience something new or exciting in your life.

To see real change, you must take real action. But sometimes, the thought of taking a massive action can seriously overwhelm us and actually prevent us from taking any action whatsoever. Sometimes it will force us back into comfort.

Which is where the second stage of this principle comes into play:

COMMIT

Before you take action, you must commit to the decision you have made.

Using our skydiving example from before, you can easily go back on your decision of skydiving by letting the excitement pass and distract yourself with something else. Or if you get too nervous, you can always just back out.

This is why commitment is so important to taking action.

Once you become committed to doing something, you put more energy and resources into accomplishing it.

So let's jump (get it?) back to our skydiving example.

Some ways of committing to skydiving would be purchasing a ticket to do the jump. You could tell your friends what you were doing and to not let you off the hook. You could give yourself a deadline.

All of the above are forms of committing to an action. They will push you to persevere when you get too scared to take action. And this can apply to any action you want to take.

It is important to remember, however, that commitment only works if you follow through.

And to follow through, you must...

ACT

Taking action is absolutely crucial to making any change. I know, I've said this about 8 million times by now. But I want you to understand how important taking action is!

Everything leading up to action is just preparation. And no matter how much preparation you have, none of it can move the needle without action.

The action phase is usually what scares us the most, because now there is a real risk of failure.

Action requires consistency to work. So if you just act one time, you're going to get very limited results (if any at all) - refer to chapter 1 for a reminder.

But consistency means you have to face fear every day. Consistency means you have to force yourself into being uncomfortable over and over again.

Consistency creates discipline and discipline creates confidence.

We could take action and fail. We could take action and get hurt. We could take action and hate ourselves.

See, this is what stops most people from action in the first place.

Unfortunately, these are the same people that spend most of their lives regretting the things they never did and blaming everyone else for why they aren't where they want to be.

I don't want this for you.

So here's your bulletproof action plan. If you follow this plan exactly as it's laid out, I promise you with 100% certainty you will get what you want out of life.

If you don't follow it, that's on you.

* * *

BULLETPROOF ACTION PLAN:

1. Define Your Goal- You can't know where you want to go or what you want to achieve if your goal is vague. Vague goals blur vision. Most people have an idea of what they want but never go much deeper than that. Spend time focusing and refining what you really want until you can see it clear as day in your mind. What does your life look like when you've reached this goal? How do you feel? What are the beliefs you have? How are you giving back to the world? This goal should inspire you and empower you to grow every time you think of it.

2. Set Your Intention- Having a goal isn't enough to inspire change. Commit to your goal by putting all of your energy into achieving it. By setting your intention, you're giving your subconscious mind a purpose. Without a strong intention, it becomes infinitely easier to lose focus in pursuit of our goals. With intention set to guide you, you will always have a direction to go even when you feel like you don't know what to do next. Practice visualizing yourself stepping into your purpose and pursuing your goal to help pull out the full power of intention.

3. Establish Your Accountability System- This can be a person, mantra, reward system, non-negotiable rules, etc. Create a dedicated form of accountability that won't let you quit when you get scared to make a big decision or things start to get tough on your way to change. Without accountability, we tend to give in to our excuses much easier than if we had someone or something to keep us on course.

4. One Percent (See previous chapter)

5. Persevere- This is the hardest part of the plan. You will be tested, beat up, challenged, confused, and so many other less desirable things on your journey towards change. If you quit when faced with these challenges, you will drive yourself deeper into comfort and you will lose belief in your ability to accomplish anything great. But if you press on through the trials, your success will get easier by the day. And, honestly, if you can master the art of perseverance, life becomes infinitely easier. Learning to persevere through anything that happens to you is what separates the truly successful from those that just can't seem to get ahead.

* * *

Seems pretty simple, right?

It's supposed to be.

We have a tendency of believing that achieving great things or making a big change in our lives takes complex, multi-faceted plans of execution.

In reality, the more complex a task is, the less likely we are to complete it.

Complexity breeds confusion. Confusion fuels doubt. Doubt kills dreams.

If you are really determined to make a change in your life, the solution lies in your ability to effectively decide what you want, commit to making it happen, and act on your commitment.

CHAPTER NINE

Principle 4: Prioritize Growth

*"Things which matter most
must never be at the mercy of
things which matter least. "
- Johann Wolfgang von Goethe*

We live our lives in accordance with our priorities. Sometimes these priorities are good for us, and sometimes they are good for other people.

Regardless, we will always find a way to meet our priorities.

This isn't such a bad thing, unless we realize that whatever we're making a priority isn't really helping us get to where we want to go.

Think of when you had to meet a deadline in a very short amount of time. Chances are you channeled all your focus and determination into meeting that deadline.

You pulled together resources, you skipped meals, you committed yourself to completing the task, and you worked harder than you ever had before just to get this task done by the deadline.

You were probably very stressed, tired, and mentally spent by the end. But you also felt a great sense of pride and accomplishment for putting yourself in a "success is the only option" situation and coming out on top.

Now, in order to actually make this happen you had to do one very specific thing.

You had to make completing the task by the deadline an absolute top priority. This is why you were successful.

You didn't allow for other distractions or responsibilities to interfere with your mission of meeting the deadline. And if there were other things that needed to be taken care of during the process, you dealt with them efficiently and only spent as much time on them as needed before returning to your work.

So how can we channel all of our energy into getting something done in such a short amount of time when making small changes in our daily habits seem impossible?

Well, pressure is definitely a helpful force in meeting a deadline. But, ultimately, it's because we made accomplishing our task our number one priority.

PRIORITY LADDER

The priority ladder is a framework I developed while I was in the middle of a half day workshop, teaching people how to rewire their brains to break free from limiting beliefs and destructive patterns.

I was working with this one woman in the crowd who really wanted to lose weight and work on her self image, but consistently failed.

After talking with her for about 10 minutes, it clicked. Her priorities were making it impossible for her to achieve her goal.

I ran to the front of the room and started drawing like a madman on a large flip chart. I wanted everyone to benefit from the lesson, even though I didn't fully understand it until it was fully drawn out in front of me.

See, we all operate in a state of cascading priorities.

Priority number one will always get your attention before priority number two. So on and so forth.

Usually, we have a "top five" list of priorities that governs our lives.

Think of these top five priorities as rungs on a ladder, with five being the bottom rung and one being the top.

So, back to the example of the woman at the workshop. We'll call her Betty.

As I was drawing the priority ladder on an oversized piece of flip chart paper, I had Betty list out her priorities for me from 1-5, with 1 being the most important and 5 being least important.

"Number 1 is definitely family," she said confidently. "Then it's work, friends, exercise, and sleep, in that order."

1. Family
2. Work
3. Friends
4. Exercise
5. Sleep

Now, this isn't a bad list of priorities. However, they were interacting in a way that was preventing her from reaching her goal.

When I asked her why dieting wasn't one of her priorities since she wanted to lose weight, she said it was; it just wasn't in the top 5.

Understand that the further down on your ladder a priority is, the less attention you will give it in day to day life.

The way the priority ladder works is we will always prioritize whatever is above a lower rung priority until it's taken care of.

For Betty, exercising was four rungs down on her priority ladder, with friends being right above it. Which do you think Betty would choose if her friends invited her out to dinner in the same time slot as when she was planning to exercise?

She would choose going to dinner with her friends, because that's a higher priority for her. And, speaking of higher priorities, do you think she would choose a healthy meal while she was out or something with more flavor and calories? (Remember, dieting is not in her top 5)

As we were further breaking down Betty's ladder, we both started to see habitual patterns that had been preventing her from making progress towards her goals as a result of her misplaced priorities.

- She would take work calls while she was out with friends.
- She kept her phone on her at the gym in case family, friends, or work needed her.
- She would lose sleep because she felt guilty for not working out, or worked out later than usual and it kept her awake.

See how these priorities all interact?

The real breakthrough came when I asked a simple question about her top priority.

I asked, "Does your family support your weight loss?"

She hesitated a moment, put her head down, and started crying.

Betty proceeded to tell me that her husband and father (who lived with her) would always give her a hard time when she would leave to go to the gym. They ate very poorly and would ridicule her if she made them a healthy meal (they were both quite capable of cooking by the way), they would often call and interrupt her while she was at the gym or out for a walk with her friends.

Since family was number one on her priority ladder, she always took their calls, cooked the food they wanted to eat, and did whatever she could to avoid being ridiculed for trying to better herself.

After we worked through a solution that empowered Betty to take full control of her ladder (read: life), many others in the workshop came forward and started telling similar stories about how other priorities actually prevented and discouraged them from even going after the things they wanted.

* * *

LIST YOUR CURRENT TOP 5 PRIORITIES:

1_____

2_____

3_____

4_____

5_____

Does that list inspire you? Is the list congruent with who you want to be and how you want to live? Can you notice any patterns or priorities that might be interfering with you living the life that you want?

If your priority ladder is not set up in a way that helps you get what you want, you will always be left feeling unfulfilled.

Create a new priority ladder right now. One that inspires you to take action and will support you in your mission each day, even when you don't feel like it.

You don't have to create an entirely different list, either. Sometimes all it takes is rearranging a few priorities to create massive change.

Here's an example. We'll use Betty's priority ladder from earlier.

Her old priority ladder was:

1. Family
2. Work
3. Friends
4. Exercise
5. Sleep

To take total control of her weight loss, we spent a good amount of time rearranging her priority ladder - not replacing - as these were all still very important priorities to her.

Betty's new priority ladder became:

1. Healthy Lifestyle (this included both exercise and diet)
2. Family
3. Work
4. Sleep
5. Friends

Now, does this new priority ladder mean she'll never make time for her family because she's working out? Or she won't ever spend time with her friends because she wants to sleep all the time?

Not in the slightest.

What this new priority ladder means is that she won't sacrifice her own growth for other people. She can learn to integrate a healthy lifestyle; even if she doesn't have support at home, she can make congruent choices while she's out. She won't answer calls in the middle of a workout.

Once the higher level priority is taken care of, she can move down the ladder. So, if she got a full night's rest the day before and knows she will be able to do the same today, she can spend time with her friends because that won't be cutting into her priority of sleep.

And, most importantly, in the event she has to climb down the ladder to tend to something that needs immediate attention, she can climb back up as soon as she's finished in order to take care of her top priority.

The key here is to set up your new priority ladder in a way that doesn't require you to add stress to your life. It should leave you feeling a sense of accomplishment and determination that no matter what comes your way, you're going to be consistently making your goals a priority.

So now, write out your new priority ladder below. Make sure it's set up in a way that assists you in moving forward. Be careful not to give yourself a priority ladder that isn't sustainable, otherwise it won't work.

NEW PRIORITY LADDER

1_____

2_____

3_____

4_____

5_____

When you were writing out the new priority ladder, did you feel excited? Could you see the opportunity that lies ahead of you if you just rearrange or add one thing to your daily operating system?

Feel free to create new priority ladders as your life begins to change. It's important to remember that not every priority that gets you to where you want to be will be a priority that will help you move past that point.

CHAPTER TEN

The Biggest Lie You Tell Yourself

"Our deepest fear is not that we are inadequate.

Our deepest fear is that we are powerful beyond measure.

It is our light, not our darkness, that most frightens us..."

-Marianne Williamson

I've been coaching people on how to take back control of their mind, body, emotional strength, and just about everything else for the past 7 years.

Every single time I sit down to a coaching session I'm filled with excitement, nervousness, confidence, and fulfillment all at once.

And I love this; I'm meant for this.

While I still have a ways to go, I'm so much further along than I was.

In fact, some of my first coaching sessions were done on park benches at my local university with anybody that would give me a chance!

Seriously, it was an interesting start to my career.

When I look back on some of the things I used to believe and methods I used to employ I could cringe.

And yet, that's what has made the journey so fun.

But there was a time when I quit.

I quit for a while.

I was struggling financially.

My coaching business was growing but not at a rate that could reliably pay my bills.

So I got a job.

Growing a business from the ground up is hard enough as it is, but throw in a full time job on top of that and you're headed for a lot of headaches and sleepless nights.

There came a point where I had to choose. Do I:

- Keep the job

or

- Focus on my coaching business

I kept the job.

It was my security. My safety net. My path of least resistance.

For the first time in over a year I didn't have to worry about making my rent payment on time. I could go to sleep at night and rest easy. I wasn't filled with the daily thoughts of "What am I going to do?"

I finally felt some semblance of peace...

.....for a little while.

- My days started getting longer.

- My attitude started getting increasingly negative.

- My health was starting to deteriorate and I began sinking into what I like to refer to as a "mini" depression.

I knew deep down that the job I was in wasn't what I wanted. I knew the life I was creating as a result of coping with the job would only lead to more problems for me down the line.

My relationships were deteriorating. I felt like I had no life outside of work. When my shift would end, all I would do is go home, sit alone, and distract myself from my reality.

The hardest part about sinking into this self-hate fueled misery was doing so with the knowledge that I *chose* this. I chose the job because I gave up on myself when my back was against the wall.

I did exactly what I would teach my clients *not* to do. I felt like a hypocrite.

My passion and purpose was to help people get out of their own way and live better lives, and I couldn't do that at my job. I had effectively traded my fulfillment in both my career and my life for some money.

All because I didn't believe I was good enough to be successful on my own.

I knew if I stayed too long in this negative state of mind I'd find myself trapped there. And one day I said enough is enough. I'd rather bet on myself and lose in my own business than completely lose myself for the sake of somebody else's.

Believing in myself was one of the most challenging decisions I ever made. And yet, it remains the most rewarding.

* * *

The biggest lie you tell yourself is "I'm not good enough."

And the more you tell yourself this, the more you'll start believing it.

Once you believe it, that becomes your truth. And, in turn, that becomes your life.

A life of never feeling good enough...

This, my friends, is the ultimate failure.

As I'm sure you've figured out by now, I'm no longer at my old job and I'm back to coaching full time. To say I've never been more at peace - even in times of high stress - is an understatement.

Having the confidence to live your life as though you have nothing to prove - to truly love yourself for everything that you are - will allow you to become whoever you want to be.

And this is why I wanted to write this book for you.

I want you to have that confidence.

I want you to live for you and give back as much as you can.

I want you to feel happy when you wake up and at peace when you rest.

I want you to feel fulfilled in your career.

I want you to have optimal health.

I want you to thrive, not just survive.

And if all you take from this book is one thing, I want it to be this:

You're already good enough. You have what it takes. You can do this.

You just have to take that first step.

CHAPTER ELEVEN

Shedding Skin

"While you are experimenting, do not remain content with the surface of things."

-Ivan Pavlov

If you're familiar with the history of psychology at all, or you just know random facts, you might recall a man by the name of Dr. Ivan Pavlov.

For those that don't know, I'll give a brief explanation.

Dr. Pavlov was a researcher interested in behavior patterns. He noticed that when dogs were presented with food, they would salivate.

The dogs salivated every single time he gave them food.

So, Dr. Pavlov had an idea. What would happen if, just before giving the dogs food, they heard a bell ring? Would it be possible to condition the same salivation response with a new trigger?

At first, nothing changed. This was to be expected.

Rings Bell > Presents Food > Dog Salivates

After repeating this sequence multiple times over, the dogs began to associate the bell ringing sound with food. So every time they heard a bell ring, the dogs would begin to salivate regardless of whether or not food was present.

Rings Bell > Dog Salivates > Presents Food

What Dr. Pavlov learned from this is that we can influence our behavior, both positively and negatively, based on what we associate pain and pleasure to. Now that the dogs knew the bell ringing sound meant food, they associated a pleasure response (saliva) when they heard the bell.

This is scientifically referred to as classical conditioning.

This one study helped paved the way for understanding human learning and behavior.

Let's explore how it interacts with you.

What have you associated personal development books to in your own conditioning?

Have they brought about a pleasure response from you - excitement, empowerment, growth, change?

Or a negative response - overwhelmed, frustrated, lacking self-confidence, disinterest?

Because right now, you're finishing a personal development book. And how you respond to this stimulus will determine the quality of your life moving forward.

Now I want you to think back on all the previous times you've read books, attended seminars, sought coaching, went to therapy, etc. Think of all the times you've tried to work on yourself in the past.

Which ones were successful?

Which ones weren't?

What was your response to all of those stimuli in the past?

Did you take what you were learning, apply it to your life, and bring about change?

Or did you just let it slide in and out of your life as though it were simply a phase?

I'm asking you this because classical conditioning tells us that when we've conditioned a response to a stimulus (in this case, how you will respond in your life as a result of reading this book), we consistently fulfill our programmed response.

In layman's terms, *if you never take action on the books you read, this is your chance to disrupt your conditioning and start responding to your life in a way that brings you massive growth, confidence, and fulfillment.*

The key difference between us humans responding to stimuli and those dogs from Dr. Pavlov's study is **choice.**

We have the ability to choose how we respond. We can choose what to do when presented with a stimulus. Choice is what separates the winners from the losers. Choice is at the fulcrum of action and excuse.

The power to choose what you do from this point forward is the greatest gift you already have available to you.

* * *

THE MOST IMPORTANT CHOICE YOU'LL EVER MAKE

Snakes shed their skin two to four times per year. This process is often referred to as molting.

The snake sheds its skin because it needs to allow for further growth.

As a snake grows, the skin begins to stretch and weaken.

This process also removes parasites that have attached themselves to the old skin.

What's interesting is that the snake's skin does not grow with the snake. Instead, a new layer of skin forms underneath the old one.

As soon as the new layer of skin is formed, the old skin begins to peel away.

What's left is a hollow shell resembling what the snake used to look like, along with all the parasites that have attached themselves to that skin.

Now, here's the most important part of this process.

If a snake does not completely shed its old skin, the secretions released by the snake during the molting process will essentially glue the old skin to the new skin.

When this happens, **the snake dies.**

If you've made it this far in the book, you've likely started to grow new skin.

You've realized new possibilities for yourself.

You've identified weaknesses and patterns that you're committed to improving.

You've gone through the painful process of getting brutally honest with yourself and where you are in life.

You've keyed in on the "parasites" that have attached themselves to you.

And now your old skin is starting to stretch.

After you finish this book, you're going to be left with a choice.

You can:

A. **Shed your old skin to make way for new growth**

B. **Let your old skin attach to the new**

And if you choose option B, remember what happens to the snake.

WANT MORE?

What kind of a coach would I be if I didn't provide you with an opportunity to continue your growth and learning now that you've already made it this far?

A bad one. I'd be a bad one.

So let's not make this our last dance.

- Follow me on Facebook and Instagram @chazmalewski

- Send me an email chaz@riseabovelifecoaching.com with the subject "I read the book!" and let's get to know each other! (I'm serious on this one. If you e-mail me, I will reply. Not an assistant. Not a bot. ME)

- Get free access to some of my best work on my website: riseabovelifecoaching.com

- I take personal coaching clients on a very limited basis. If you're interested in coaching, please send me an email at the address provided above with the subject line "Coaching."

CPSIA information can be obtained
at www.ICGtesting.com
Printed in the USA
BVHW060118020321
601389BV00007B/997